Breathing Easy

Your Essential Guide to Understanding, Preventing COPD, Lung Cancer, FLU, Asthma, Pneumonia, Chest Pain, and Pulmonary Embolism

Dr. Louisa Jenkins

Copyright @2024

The content in this book is for general informational purposes only and is not meant to be medical advice. Its objective is to support and educate readers who are interested in learning more about lung disorders and how to manage them. It is advisable for readers to seek the advice of licensed medical professionals for personalized lung disease diagnosis, treatment, and management.

The author or publisher does not support or advocate any particular medical treatments, goods, or services; all references to such are made for informational purposes only. Before making any medical decisions, readers are urged to do their own research and speak with medical professionals.

Table of Contents

Chapter One

Introduction

This book can be helpful whether you are providing care for a sick person, have a lung condition yourself, or are simply interested in learning more about how to better take care of your lungs. Any ailment that affects the lungs and prevents them from functioning normally is considered a lung illness. Lung disease can strike anyone at any time. Men, women, kids, smokers, ex-smokers, and never-smokers should all receive the same level of support and respect.

The primary and most complex respiratory organ, the lungs, expand and contract hundreds of times a day in order to take in oxygen and release carbon dioxide. Because our lungs are an essential organ for breathing, we must take good care of them. Since the lungs are susceptible to various infections and abnormalities, lung diseases rank among the world's top causes of death.

Among the most prevalent medical disorders worldwide are lung ailments. Lung disease affects tens of millions of people in the United States alone. Lung issues are mostly caused by three factors: heredity, smoking, and infections.

As part of an intricate system, your lungs expand and contract hundreds of times a day to take in oxygen and release carbon dioxide. Any issue pertaining to any component of this system could result in lung disease.

There are three primary categories of lung diseases:

- **Airway diseases:** The tubes, or airways, that convey gases other than oxygen into and out of the lungs are impacted by a number of disorders. They typically result in a narrowing or obstruction of the airways. Asthma, bronchiolitis, bronchiectasis, and chronic obstructive pulmonary disease (COPD), which is the main ailment affecting individuals with cystic fibrosis, are the examples of airway ailments. Symptoms of respiratory disorders are often described by sufferers as "trying to breathe out through a straw."

- **Lung tissue diseases**: Lung tissue's structural integrity is impacted by several illnesses. In restrictive lung disease, the lungs' capacity to expand to their maximum extent is restricted by tissue inflammation or scarring. The lungs so have difficulty taking in oxygen and exhaling carbon dioxide. Many individuals suffering with this kind of lung disease describes feeling as though they are "wearing a too-tight sweater or vest." They are consequently unable to inhale deeply. Sarcoidosis and pulmonary fibrosis are examples of lung tissue diseases.

Lung circulation diseases: The lungs' blood arteries are impacted by these illnesses. They are brought on by blood vessel irritation, scarring, or clotting. They have an impact on the lungs' capacity to absorb oxygen and expel carbon dioxide. Some illnesses may have an impact on how well the heart functions. Pulmonary hypertension is one disorder that affects the circulation in the lungs. When they exert themselves, people with these diseases frequently experience severe dyspnea.

Chapter Two

Common Lung Diseases

As a group, diseases of the lungs, lung tissue, and lung circulation fall under the umbrella term "lung disease," some of which are capable of leading to respiratory failure. Asthma, pneumonia, influenza, pulmonary embolism, and tuberculosis are among the ailments listed here.

Asthma

When you have asthma, your airways narrow, widen, and may produce more mucus. Coughing, dyspnea, and wheezing upon exhalation could be symptoms of breathing issues.

Asthma is merely a minor discomfort for some people. For others, it could be a serious issue that makes life challenging and raises the risk of a deadly asthma attack.

Although asthma cannot be cured, its symptoms can be managed. Since asthma frequently fluctuates over time, it's critical that you and your doctor monitor your symptoms and modify your treatment strategy as necessary.

Symptoms

The symptoms of asthma vary from person to person. While some people have symptoms only sometimes, like during an asthma attack, others may experience symptoms constantly.

Among the signs and symptoms of asthma are:

- Breathlessness
- Chest tightness or pain wheezing during exhalation, which is frequently a symptom of childhood asthma coughing, wheezing, or dyspnea that keeps you from falling asleep
- episodes of respiratory distress, such as a cold or flu-like illness, that worsen coughing or wheezing.

The following are signs that your asthma is probably becoming worse:

- Symptoms and indicators of asthma that are annoying and increasingly prevalent include breathing becoming more difficult, as seen by a peak flow meter, a tool that measures lung function.

- The requirement to regularly use a quick-relief inhaler

Some persons experience flare-ups of their asthma symptoms and warning indicators in specific situations:

- In cold, dry air, asthma triggered by exercise may worsen.
- Allergies-induced asthma brought on by airborne pollutants such as mold spores, pollen, cockroach excrement, or animal dander—dry saliva released by pets—or skin pieces occupational asthma brought on by dust, fumes, chemicals, or other allergens at work

When to see a doctor

- It is possible for asthma attacks to be lethal. Decide whether you should see a doctor straight immediately and what to do if your symptoms get worse in consultation with your doctor. An asthma episode can cause symptoms such as:

- wheeze or dyspnea that worsens quickly
- Not even with an inhaler for quick relief from respiratory issues when engaging in moderate exercise
- See your doctor if you experience any other symptoms of asthma, such as a persistent cough or continuous wheezing that lasts more than a few days. Early asthma treatment reduces lung damage over time and stops the condition from getting worse.
- Asthma sufferers should collaborate with their physician to manage their symptoms. Sufficient long-term care not only improves quality of life on a daily basis but also averts potentially lethal asthma episodes.
- If, in spite of your medicine, your symptoms don't seem to be improving or if you need to use your quick-relief inhaler more frequently, you should see

your doctor right once. Never take more medication than is recommended without first consulting your doctor. Overusing asthma medication might have unanticipated negative effects and exacerbate your asthma.

- Asthma frequently evolves over time. Schedule regular check-ups with your doctor so you can discuss any necessary therapy adjustments and describe your symptoms.

Causes of Asthma

While the precise etiology of asthma remains unknown, a combination of environmental and inherited factors is most likely to blame.

Asthma triggers

Exposure to allergens and other irritants might result in asthma symptoms and signs. The things that induce asthma vary from person to person and can include:

- Airborne allergens include dust mites, mold spores, pollen, pet dander, and cockroach dung particles.

- respiratory ailments, such a common cold
- Engage in cold air exercise
- Smoke and other air pollutants and irritants
- ibuprofen and naproxen sodium (Advil, Motrin IB, and other brands), as well as beta blockers and aspirin, are examples of nonsteroidal anti-inflammatory medicines (NSAIDs) (Aleve)
- Fear and intense feelings
- Certain foods and beverages, such as shrimp, dried fruit, processed potatoes, beer, and wine, include additional sulfites and preservatives.
- Acid reflux from the stomach refluxes into the throat, a condition known as reflux disease (GERD).

Risk factors

- Many variables are known to raise your risk of acquiring asthma. These include: having a brother or parent with asthma in your biological family; having another allergic reaction, including atopic dermatitis, which results in red, itchy skin; or having hay fever, which causes runny nose, congestion, and itchy eyes.

- Smoking, being overweight, and being around secondhand smoke
- exposure to exhaust fumes from other sources of pollution or contaminants exposure to substances used in industry, agriculture, and hair salons as occupational triggers

Complications

- Asthma-related complications include of the following:
- symptoms that make it difficult to work, sleep, or perform other chores
- days absent from work or school due to asthma attacks
- chronic constriction of the bronchial tube, a tube that transports air to and from your lungs and impairs breathing
- severe asthma episodes necessitating ER visits and hospital stays

- adverse effects of several drugs taken over time to treat severe asthma
- The prevention of asthma's short- and long-term effects depends heavily on receiving the right care.

Chronic obstructive pulmonary disease (COPD)

Chronic obstructive pulmonary disease (COPD) is a chronic inflammatory lung condition that results in limited lung airflow. Wheezing, coughing up mucus (sputum), and breathing difficulty are some of the symptoms. It is typically brought on by prolonged contact to irritant chemicals or particulate matter, most frequently from smoking cigarettes. Heart disease, lung cancer, and a host of other ailments are more common in those with COPD.

COPD is mostly caused by two basic diseases: emphysema and chronic bronchitis. People with COPD typically have both of these illnesses at the same time; however, their severity can vary.

The lining of the bronchial tubes, which transport air to and from the lungs' alveoli, becomes inflamed when someone has chronic bronchitis. Sputum (mucus) discharge and a daily cough are its defining characteristics.

Emphysema is a condition that arises from damage to the lungs' alveoli, which are tiny airways at the end of the lungs called bronchioles, caused by nicotine smoke and other irritating chemicals and particles.

Despite being a progressive disorder that deteriorates with time, COPD is curable. Most COPD patients can obtain good symptom control, a high quality of life, and a lower chance of developing other related disorders with appropriate therapy.

Symptoms

The signs and symptoms of COPD typically take longer to manifest, especially if smoking exposure persists, and they frequently do not become apparent until considerable lung damage has occurred.

Listed below are a few COPD symptoms and indicators:

breathing issues, especially when moving about

Wheezing, chest tightness, clear, white, yellow, or greenish mucus respiratory tract infections, or persistent cough that may generate sputum energy deficiency unintentional weight loss (in later stages)

edema in the legs, foot, or ankles

A period of several days or more, known as an exacerbation, is when a person with COPD suffers symptoms that are more severe than they typically are on a daily basis.

When to see a doctor

Speak with your doctor if your symptoms do not go better or get worse after therapy, or if you experience any infection-related symptoms like fever or changes in your sputum.

If you have any of the following symptoms: rapid heartbeat, dyspnea, vertigo, difficulty concentrating, or a significant blueness of the lips or nail beds (cyanosis), get medical help right once.

Causes

Tobacco usage is the primary cause of COPD in developed nations. People who live in poorer countries with poor ventilation and who are exposed to fuel pollution from cooking and heating are at high risk of developing COPD.

While many smokers with long smoking histories may have impaired lung function, only a small percentage of long-term smokers acquire clinically evident COPD. Certain smokers have a lower incidence of lung problems. They can receive an incorrect diagnosis of COPD if a more comprehensive evaluation is not performed.

How your lungs are affected

Your lungs receive air through two sizable tubes known as the trachea, sometimes known as the windpipe (bronchi). Your lungs' main tubes split into several smaller tubes, or bronchioles, which ultimately congregate into clusters of microscopic air sacs known as alveoli, which resemble tree branches.

Many microscopic blood arteries are located within the extremely thin walls of the air sacs, also known as capillaries. As you breathe in, oxygen from the surrounding air enters your body through these blood vessels. Carbon dioxide, a waste product of metabolism, is simultaneously exhaled.

To expel air from your body, your lungs rely on the suppleness of the bronchial tubes and air sacs. They become less elastic and overexpand as a result of COPD, which means that some of the air you exhale becomes stuck in your lungs.

Causes of airway obstruction

The following are some causes of blockage of the airways:

Cigarette smoke and other irritants: Long-term tobacco smoking is the primary cause of lung damage for most COPD patients. Since not everyone who smokes gets COPD, there may be additional factors at work as well, like a hereditary predisposition to the disease.

Air pollution, secondhand smoke, pipe smoke, cigar smoke, and exposure to dust, smoke, or fumes at work are additional irritants that may aggravate COPD.

Emphysema: The delicate alveolar walls and elastic fibers are destroyed by this lung disease. When you exhale, your small airways shrink, making it harder for air to leave your lungs.

Chronic bronchitis: This illness can further obstruct the airways in addition to producing more mucus in the lungs, inflaming the bronchial tubes, and narrowing them. You start hacking in an attempt to get your airways clear.

Alpha-1-antitrypsin deficiency: Due to a genetic condition known as alpha-1-antitrypsin deficiency (AAt), about 1% of COPD patients have low disease levels. To help shield the lungs, the liver makes and releases AAt into the bloodstream. Liver illness, lung disease, or both can result from a lack of alpha-1-antitrypsin.

Adults with COPD associated with AAt deficiency can get treatment options that are comparable to those offered to patients with more prevalent forms of COPD. Furthermore, part of the treatment occasionally entails replacing the absent at protein, which may stop additional lung damage.

Risk factors

The risk factors for COPD include:

- **Exposure to tobacco smoke:** A history of continuous cigarette smoking is the main risk factor for COPD. Your risk increases with the number of years you've smoked and your age. People who use tobacco products, like cigars, pipes, marijuana, or who are frequently around secondhand smoke may also be at risk.

- **People with asthma:** A long-term inflammatory respiratory condition called asthma may increase the chance of getting COPD. Asthma and smoking together significantly increase the risk of COPD development.

- **Exposure to dusts and chemicals:** At work, prolonged exposure to chemical vapors, fumes, or dusts can cause irritation and inflammation of the lungs.
- **Exposure to fuel fumes:** Living in homes with inadequate ventilation and being near fuel emissions from cooking and heating puts people in developing nations at higher risk of developing COPD.
- **Genetics:** A rare genetic condition called alpha-1-antitrypsin deficiency is linked to certain cases of COPD. Due to a higher number of hereditary hazards, smokers have a higher chance of developing the condition.

Complications

COPD can lead to a number of issues, such as:

- **Respiratory infections:** Colds, the flu, and pneumonia are more common in people with COPD.

Breathing becomes considerably more difficult and lung tissue damage can worsen with any respiratory infection.

- **Heart issues:** For unknown reasons, having COPD may make you more susceptible to heart issues, such as a heart attack.

- **Lung cancer:** The risk of lung cancer is increased in people with COPD.

- **High blood pressure in the arteries supplying blood to the lungs**: One potential effect of COPD is pulmonary hypertension, or elevated blood pressure in these arteries.

- **Depression:** If you have breathing problems, you could find it difficult to engage in enjoyable activities. Furthermore, dealing with a major sickness may result in depression.

Lung Cancer

One kind of cancer that starts in the lungs is lung cancer. The two spongy tissues in your chest, your lungs, are responsible for exhaling carbon dioxide and absorbing oxygen.

Globally, lung cancer is the primary cause of cancer-related deaths.

Smokers are more likely to develop lung cancer than non-smokers, but lung cancer can still strike anyone. You have a higher chance of developing lung cancer the longer you have smoked cigarettes. Even if you have smoked for a long time, you will greatly reduce your chance of lung cancer if you give up.

Symptoms

In its early stages, lung cancer usually shows no symptoms at all. Lung cancer usually shows signs and symptoms after the disease has progressed.

Some indications and symptoms of lung cancer include the following:

- a chronic cough that just now began to produce blood, even a tiny bit of it

- Out of breath
- chest ache
- loud, sibilant voice
- Being physically fit without straining oneself or experiencing bone discomfort
- A headache

When to see a doctor

If you're concerned about any persistent signs or symptoms, schedule an appointment with your doctor.

If you smoke and have not been able to successfully stop, schedule a visit with your doctor. Your physician can provide advice on how to stop smoking, as well as prescription medications, therapy that substitutes nicotine, and counseling.

Causes of Lung Cancer

Lung cancer is mostly caused by smoking in both smokers and those who have been exposed to secondhand smoke. However, it is possible for someone who has never smoked or who has never spent a substantial amount of time around secondhand smoke to develop lung cancer. There are situations where lung cancer has no known cause.

How lung cancer is caused by smoking

Medical professionals claim that smoking increases the risk of lung cancer by destroying the cells lining the lungs. Inhaled cigarette smoke, a mixture of chemicals known as carcinogens that cause cancer, quickly alters lung tissue.

Your body might be able to repair this injury at first. However, the good cells lining your lungs get more harmed with each exposure. Damage to cells over time can result in aberrant behavior that could eventually lead to cancer.

Types of lung cancer

Based on the microscopic morphology of the cancer cells, doctors divide lung cancer patients into two main types. Your primary form of lung cancer will determine the best course of treatment for you, as determined by your doctor.

Two main forms of lung cancer can be identified:

- **Small cell lung cancer:** Almost mainly affecting heavy smokers, small cell lung cancer is less common than non-small cell lung cancer.
- **Non-small cell lung cancer:** Numerous subtypes of lung cancer are included in this general phrase. Adenocarcinoma, large cell carcinoma, and squamous cell carcinoma are examples of non-small cell lung malignancies.

Risk factors

There are more variables that could increase your risk of developing lung cancer. It is possible to control some risk factors, including stopping smoking. Furthermore, you have no influence over certain circumstances, such as your family history.

Risk factors for lung cancer include:

- Taking tobacco
- Being near someone smoking
- Previous radiotherapy
- Having been exposed to radon
- exposure to other toxins and asbestos

- A history of lung cancer in the family

Complications

Lung cancer may result in the following effects:

- **Shortness of breath:** Dyspnea in lung cancer patients occurs when the malignant tumor is so big that it blocks one or more main airways. Moreover, fluid buildup around the lungs caused by lung cancer may inhibit the afflicted lung from fully extending when breathing.

- **Coughing up blood:** Lung cancer can cause hemoptysis, or bleeding in the airways, which is why you could cough up blood. Severe bleeding does occur occasionally. There are treatments available to stop bleeding.

- **Pain:** Pain could result from advanced lung cancer if it spreads to the lung lining or to another part of the body, including the bone. Inform your physician if you have any discomfort; there are various methods to manage pain.

- **Fluid in the chest (pleural effusion):** The area of the chest cavity surrounding the wounded lung, known as the pleural space, may become inundated with fluid due to lung cancer. Dyspnea may be brought on by an accumulation of fluid in the chest. There are ways to relax the pressure in your chest and lessen the chance of developing another pleural effusion.

- **Cancer that metastasizes:** When lung cancer spreads, it typically affects other organs like the brain and bones. Depending on which organ is impacted, cancer that spreads can produce discomfort, nausea, headaches, or other symptoms. Lung cancer is usually incurable once it has spread to other parts of the body. You can live a longer life and have your symptoms reduced with the help of treatments.

Pneumonia

An infection that inflames one or both of the lung's air sacs is known as pneumonia. Fever, chills, dyspnea, and a productive cough with purulent material can all be symptoms of the air sacs filling with fluid or pus. Pneumonia can be caused by a wide range of species, including bacteria, viruses, and fungus.

The severity of pneumonia can vary from moderate to fatal. The most susceptible include children under five, people over 65, people with compromised immune systems, and people who are ill.

Symptoms

Your age, general health, and the type of germ that caused the illness will all influence how severe your pneumonia symptoms are. Minor symptoms and indicators can occasionally be confused for flu or cold symptoms, even if they last longer.

Some indications and symptoms of pneumonia include the following:

- chest pain while inhalation or coughing

- Perplexing or changed states of awareness (in those 65 years of age and older)
- a potentially mucus-producing cough
- Sweating, chills, and exhaustion fever
- a body temperature that is below normal (in people over 65 and immune system compromised persons)
- diarrhea, vomiting, or nausea
- Breathlessness

It's possible for newborns and infants to display no symptoms at all. Along with these symptoms, children may throw up, cough, have trouble breathing, or have a temperature. They might also seem agitated, exhausted, or devoid of vitality. It's possible for newborns and infants to display no symptoms at all. Along with these symptoms, children may throw up, cough, have trouble breathing, or have a temperature. They might also seem agitated, exhausted, or devoid of vitality.

When to see a doctor

Consult your physician if you get dyspnea, chest pain, a persistent cough that won't go away (102 F or higher), or difficulties breathing. (Particularly if it's creating pus).

People who fall into these high-risk categories should see a doctor in particular:

- Adults who are over 65
- Youngsters who exhibit symptoms and indicators before becoming two years old
- People who are undergoing chemotherapy or taking immune-suppressive drugs, or who have underlying medical conditions

In certain old people, heart failure patients, and anyone with long-term lung issues, pneumonia can rapidly become a life-threatening illness.

Causes

Pneumonia can be caused by several different microbes. Airborne pollutants mostly consist of viruses and bacteria. Usually, the illness that these microorganisms are producing in your lungs is eliminated by your body. Even though everything about your health is fine overall, there are instances when these pathogens overwhelm your immune system.

The classification of pneumonia is based on the kinds of bacteria that cause the sickness as well as the site of infection.

Community-acquired pneumonia

The most prevalent kind of pneumonia is community-acquired pneumonia. It takes place outside of hospitals and other healthcare facilities. It could result from:

- **Bacteria:** The most frequent cause of bacterial pneumonia in the United States is streptococcus pneumoniae. This kind of pneumonia can develop on its own or coincide with a cold or flu episode. Lobar pneumonia is the term for the condition that affects only one lung lobe.

- **Bacteria-like Organism**: Another pathogen that can cause pneumonia is Mycoplasma pneumoniae. The symptoms are typically not as severe as they can be for other types of pneumonia. The term "walking pneumonia" is occasionally used to describe this kind of pneumonia because it usually doesn't necessitate bed rest.

- **Fungi:** Individuals with compromised immune systems, chronic illnesses, and high exposure to airborne microorganisms are more susceptible to this type of pneumonia. Depending on the area, the fungus that causes it might be found in soil or bird droppings.

- **Viruses:** Numerous viruses that also cause colds and the flu can cause pneumonia. The most common cause of pneumonia in children under five is viral infection. Most cases of viral pneumonia are not very dangerous. However, things can occasionally get very serious.

Hospital-acquired pneumonia

Pneumonia can strike patients who are hospitalized for another condition. Because the germs that cause hospital-acquired pneumonia may be more resistant to medication and the patients are already ill, the condition can be dangerous. The risk of developing this kind of pneumonia is higher in patients using ventilators, or breathing machines, which are frequently seen in intensive care units.

Health care-acquired pneumonia

Healthcare-acquired pneumonia is a bacterial infection that can strike patients receiving treatment at outpatient clinics, such as renal dialysis centers, or living in long-term care homes. Similar to hospital-acquired pneumonia, healthcare-acquired pneumonia may also be brought on by drug-resistant microbes.

Aspiration pneumonia

Aspiration pneumonia may arise from inhaling liquids, food particles, vomit, or saliva into the lungs. If you suffer from a medical condition that affects your usual gag reflex, such as a brain injury, swallowing issues, or heavy alcohol or drug use, you run the risk of aspirating.

Risk factors

Anyone can contract pneumonia. However, the two age groups most at danger are those 65 years of age or older and young children. Other risk factors include:

- being transported to the medical facility
- persistent illness
- Tobacco use decreased or inhibited immunity

Complications

Some patients with pneumonia, particularly those in high-risk groups, may have side effects even after receiving therapy, such as:

- bacteria in the bloodstream (bacteremia)
- breathing difficulties
- The accumulation of fluid around the lungs, or pleural effusion, and
- Lung abscess

Pulmonary Embolism

A blood clot that obstructs and prevents blood flow to a lung artery is known as a pulmonary embolism. The blood clot typically begins in a deep vein in the leg and moves to the lung. On rare occasions, the clot could develop in a vein in some other body area. Deep vein thrombosis (DVT) is the term used to describe the formation of a blood clot in one or more deep veins throughout the body.

Pulmonary embolism can be fatal because the blood supply to the lungs is being blocked by one or more clots. Nonetheless, the chance of dying is significantly decreased with early care. By taking precautions against leg blood clots, you can lower your risk of suffering a pulmonary embolism.

Symptoms

Depending on the size of the clots, the extent of lung involvement, and whether you have any underlying heart or lung issues, pulmonary embolism symptoms can vary greatly.

Typical signs and symptoms include of:

- **Shortness of breath:** Usually, this symptom manifests abruptly. Breathing issues occur even while you're at rest and get worse with movement.

- **Chest Pain:** It can indicate that you're experiencing a heart attack. When you take a deep breath, you frequently feel and perceive pain. The pain may make it difficult for you to take deep breaths. Additionally, it could hurt when you bend, cough, or lean over.
- **Fainting:** If your blood pressure or heart rate drops suddenly, you can pass out. We call this syncope.

Additional signs and symptoms of a pulmonary embolism include:

- a cough that could discharge blood-stained or streaked mucus; a fast or erratic heartbeat
- feeling faint or lightheaded profuse sweating
- Fever Cyanosis, or discolored or clammy skin Leg discomfort or edema, commonly in the back of the lower leg, or both

When to see a doctor

A pulmonary embolism has the potential to pose a major threat to life. If you get unexpected shortness of breath, chest pain, or fainting, get medical help right once.

Causes

A pulmonary embolism can occur when a foreign substance, usually a blood clot, becomes lodged in a lung artery and obstructs blood flow. The most prevalent cause of blood clots is deep vein thrombosis, which affects the legs' deep veins.

Numerous clots are implicated in numerous cases. Every obstructed artery causes the lung tissue it supplies to lose blood flow and possibly die. One example of this is a pulmonary infarction. As a result, your lungs have a harder time supplying the rest of your body with oxygen.

Blood clots are not always the cause of blockages in blood vessels. Other possible explanations consist of:

- Within the fat of a broken long bone
- a section of the cancer
- air bubbles

Risk Factors

Although anyone can get a blood clot that results in a pulmonary embolism, there are a number of variables that could increase your risk.

- **History of blood clot**: If you or any blood relatives—a parent or sibling, for example—have ever experienced a pulmonary embolism or venous blood clot, you are more vulnerable.
- **Smoking:** Smoking raises the risk of blood clots in certain persons for unclear reasons, especially in those with additional risk factors.
- **Being overweight:** Blood clot risk is increased by being overweight, especially in those with additional risk factors.
- **Supplemental estrogen:** Birth control pills and hormone replacement treatment contain estrogen, which may raise blood clotting factors, particularly in smokers and obese people.

- **Pregnancy:** The baby's weight is pressing against the pelvic veins, which may impede the flow of blood back into the legs. When blood slows down or pools, clots are more likely to occur.

Complications

A pulmonary embolism has the potential to pose a major threat to life. The mortality rate from untreated pulmonary embolisms is around one-third. That figure, however, falls significantly if the illness is identified and treated quickly.

Another complication of pulmonary embolisms is pulmonary hypertension, or unusually high blood pressure in the lungs and right side of the heart. Your heart has to work harder to pump blood through blockages in the arteries that lead to your lungs. Over time, the excessive blood pressure weakens your heart.

Occasionally, tiny clots known as emboli stay in the lungs and cause the pulmonary arteries to deteriorate over time. Chronic pulmonary hypertension is the result of this blood flow restriction.

Tuberculosis

The serious disease known as tuberculosis (TB) mostly attacks the lungs. One specific type of bacteria is the one that causes tuberculosis.

An infected person can spread the illness by sneezing, coughing, or singing. Small amounts of the germs may be released into the air as a result of this. The bacterium can then enter someone else's lungs when they inhale the droplets.

Everywhere people congregate in large groups or live closely together, tuberculosis is known to spread. Individuals with compromised immune systems, such as those afflicted with HIV/AIDS, are more susceptible to tuberculosis than healthy individuals.

Antibiotic-containing medications are used to treat TB. However, a number of bacterial species are now resistant to certain antibiotics.

Symptoms

An infection results from the growth and multiplication of tuberculosis (TB) germs in the lungs. A TB infection progresses through three stages. Every step has a distinct set of symptoms.

Primary TB infection: The initial stage is referred to as the "main infection". Cells of the immune system locate and apprehend the invaders. The pathogens may be totally eradicated by the immune system. However, certain bacteria may manage to stay contained and grow.

An initial infection usually shows no symptoms at all in most cases. Some people may have symptoms similar to the flu, such as mild temperature, coughing, and exhaustion.

Latent TB infection: Latent tuberculosis infection is the stage that usually follows primary infection. TBC microorganisms cause immune system cells to seal off lung tissue. If the immune system manages to contain the bacteria, they will be unable to cause any further damage. The microorganisms are still there, though. When a tuberculosis infection is latent, there are no symptoms.

Active TB disease: When an infection surpasses the immune system's ability to combat it, active tuberculosis disease develops. Infections in the lungs and other body regions are brought on by germs. Active tuberculosis may arise following a primary infection. However, it typically occurs months or years following a latent tuberculosis infection.

Lung symptoms from active tuberculosis usually get worse over a few weeks. These could include symptoms like a cough, blood or mucus spitting, a chest ache, coughing up blood, fever, chills, night sweats, decreased weight, appetite refusal, exhaustion, and an overall feeling of being unwell.

Active TB disease outside the lungs: The body is capable of acquiring tuberculosis (TB) outside of the lungs. Extrapulmonary tuberculosis is the term for this. The bodily component that is infected affects the symptoms. Fever, chills, nocturnal sweats, appetite suppression, weight loss, tiredness, widespread malaise, and discomfort near the infection site are common signs and symptoms.

Although active tuberculosis in the voice box is unrelated to lung disease, its symptoms are more like to pulmonary conditions.

When to see a doctor

Many different conditions share similarities with the symptoms of TB. If, even after relaxing for a few days, your symptoms don't get better, see your doctor.

Seek immediate medical attention if any of the following symptoms apply to you: a sudden, severe headache, a stabbing pain in your chest, dizziness, convulsions, trouble breathing, or blood in your stools or urine.

Causes

Mycobacterium tuberculosis is the name of the microorganism that causes tuberculosis.

People who have active tuberculosis in their voice box or lungs can spread the illness to other people. The microscopic droplets that the bacteria emit cause them to spread throughout the atmosphere. They may cough, talk, sing, sneeze, laugh, or do any of these things. Inhaling the droplets can cause infection in a person.

People who spend more time indoors are more likely to have the illness spread. Consequently, environments where individuals live or work together for extended periods of time are more susceptible to the disease's transmission. Moreover, the illness spreads more quickly in large groups.

A latent tuberculosis infection prevents the disease from spreading to other individuals. After two to three weeks of treatment, a patient with active tuberculosis usually is not able to entirely recover from the infection.

Drug-resistant TB

Antibiotic-resistant strains of the TB bacterium have been identified. Drugs that once addressed the illness no longer function as a result.

This is partially explained by genetic alterations that bacteria naturally undergo. Unintentionally, a bacterium may acquire a trait that fortifies its resistance to an antibiotic assault. It is capable of proliferating if it survives.

More resistant strains of the bacteria can grow and thrive in situations where antibiotics are not administered correctly or do not completely eradicate the bacterium for any other reason. A new strain of the bacteria that is resistant to drugs may eventually proliferate if it spreads to other individuals.

Risk factors

Although tuberculosis can infect anyone, several variables make infection more likely. The possibility that an infection may develop into an active case of tuberculosis is increased by other factors.

If you have active TB disease or are at risk of contracting an infection, the Centers for Disease Control and Prevention advise getting tested for the condition. If you fit any of the following risk factors, speak with your healthcare physician.

Influenza (FLU)

The flu, commonly known as influenza, is a type of respiratory infection that mostly affects the lungs, nose, and throat. A virus is responsible for the flu. There is a difference between stomach "flu" viruses, which cause vomiting and diarrhea, and influenza, which is more popularly recognized as the flu.

Most influenza patients recover on their own. On the other hand, influenza and its aftereffects can occasionally be lethal. Certain populations are more vulnerable than others to complications from influenza, including:

- tiny ones, particularly those that are younger than a year.
- individuals who are contemplating a pregnancy, just gave birth, or are already pregnant during flu season.
- individuals above 65.

- those who are employed or reside in buildings housing a large number of other people.

Anybody who fits into one of the other high-risk categories for flu complications below:

- weakened defense mechanisms.
- a BMI (body mass index) of 40 or higher.
- illnesses that affect the neurological system or alter how information is processed in the brain.

In addition, an individual's chance of experiencing complications from the flu is increased by the following medical conditions:

- persons with chronic illnesses such diabetes, asthma, kidney disease, liver disease, and heart disease.
- folks who have suffered from strokes.
- those under 20 who have been taking aspirin for an extended period of time.

The annual influenza vaccination reduces the chance of developing severe flu-related symptoms, notwithstanding its modest efficacy. This is particularly true for those who are more likely to experience serious complications from the flu.

Symptoms

Flu symptoms, like runny nose, sneezing, and sore throat, can initially seem like cold symptoms. Most colds begin slowly at first. But the disease usually strikes quickly and severely. Furthermore, although a cold may cause discomfort, a flu typically worsens your symptoms.

Common flu symptoms include fever, chills, sweats, and aching muscles; however, these are not always present.

Additional signs and symptoms consist of:

- headache.
- prolonged dry cough.
- breathlessness.
- fatigue and weakness.
- congestion or nasal discharge.
- painful throat.
- eyes that hurt.

Other flu symptoms include vomiting and diarrhea. But compared to adults, youngsters are more likely to have them.

When to see a doctor

When they have the flu, most people can take care of themselves at home and don't always need to visit a doctor.

See your doctor at away if you have flu-like symptoms and there's a danger they could get worse. Antiviral medications can hasten the recovery from the flu and protect you from more serious complications.

Seek immediate medical attention if your flu symptoms are severe. Adults who experience emergency symptoms may exhibit dyspnea or dyspnea in their breathing.

- chest pains.
- vertigo and seizures.
- degradation of the underlying illnesses.
- extreme muscle pain or weakness.

Causes

Viruses are what cause influenza. When an infected individual coughs, sneezes, or speaks, the virus is released into the air in the form of droplets. The rains are instantly inhaled. Alternatively, after coming into contact with an object like a computer keyboard, the germs may enter your body through your mouth, nose, or eyes. One day before symptoms develop or up to five or seven days after they do, a person infected with the virus may be able to spread to others. Illness may spread more slowly in young people and individuals with compromised immune systems.

New strains of influenza viruses are frequently created, and the virus itself is always evolving. Should you have previously contracted influenza, your body has already produced antibodies to combat that particular strain of the virus.

These antibodies may be able to prevent infection or diminish its severity if subsequent influenza viruses are similar to ones, you have already encountered, either through personal experience with the illness or vaccination.

Conversely, antibody levels could decrease over time. Additionally, you could not be protected against newly developing influenza strains by antibodies against older influenza viruses. It is feasible for recently evolved strains to differ significantly from more established ones.

Risk factors

The following factors could make you more susceptible to contracting the flu or its complications:

- **Age:** Children younger than one year old are more vulnerable to the negative effects of seasonal influenza. Furthermore, the results are typically worse for those over 65.

- **Living or working conditions:** Flu infections are more common in people who work or reside in high-density settings, such as assisted care homes. Residents of hospitals are also more vulnerable.

- **Immune system weakness:** The immune system can be weakened by HIV/AIDS, anti-rejection medications, long-term steroid usage, organ transplants, blood cancer, and cancer treatment. This might increase the likelihood of problems and promote the spread of the flu virus.

- **Chronic illnesses:** Chronic illness sufferers can be more vulnerable to influenza-related complications. A history of stroke, lung ailments related to asthma, diabetes, heart disease, neurological disorders, metabolic abnormalities, respiratory issues, and issues involving the kidneys, liver, or blood are a few examples.

- **Race/ethnicity:** Individuals who identify as Black, Latino, American Indian, or Alaska Native may be more susceptible to influenza-related complications in the US.

- **Under-20 age group aspirin use:** Individuals under the age of twenty who are on long-term aspirin therapy and have an influenza virus infection may develop Reye's syndrome.
- **Pregnancy:** Influenza-related problems are more common in pregnant women, especially in the second and third trimesters of their pregnancy. For up to two weeks following the baby's birth, there is still a risk.
- **Obesity:** If a person's body mass index (BMI) is 40 or higher, they are more likely to experience complications from the flu.

Complications

The flu usually doesn't represent a serious threat if you're young and healthy. When you have the flu, it normally goes away in a week or two, despite how horrible it may feel. On the other hand, high-risk individuals and children may have issues like:

- Attacks of asthma

- heart problems and pneumonia

- infections in the ears

- Acute respiratory distress syndrome (bronchitis).

One of the most dangerous side effects is pneumonia. Pneumonia in the elderly and those with long-term ailments can be fatal.

Prevention of Asthma

While there is no way to prevent asthma attacks, you and your doctor can create a detailed strategy to manage your illness and prevent attacks.

- **Follow your asthma action plan:** Create a detailed strategy with your physician and the medical staff for taking your medication and controlling an asthma attack. After that, be careful to carry out your plan. Since asthma is a chronic illness, it requires constant care and observation. You may feel more in control of your life if you are in charge of your medical care.

- **Get vaccinated for influenza and pneumonia:** Maintaining up-to-date vaccination records helps stop asthma flare-ups brought on by the flu and pneumonia.

- **Find and stay away from asthma triggers:** Asthma episodes can be brought on by a variety of environmental allergens and irritants, such as mold, pollen, cold air, and air pollution. Ascertain what triggers or aggravates your asthma, then take precautions to avoid those things.

- **Keep an eye on your breathing**: You might become skilled at identifying the warning indicators of an attack, such as wheezing, dyspnea, or light coughing. However, utilize a home peak flow meter on a regular basis to measure and record your peak airflow, as your lung function may degrade before you have any symptoms or signs. Using a peak flow meter, you may gauge how hard you can exhale. You can learn how to measure your peak flow at home from your doctor.

- **Identify and treat attacks early:** Your odds of having a serious attack are decreased if you take immediate action. Additionally, you won't require as much medicine to manage your symptoms. Take your medication as directed when your peak flow values drop and warn you of an impending attack. Additionally, cease doing everything that might have sparked the assault right away. See a doctor if, despite doing what is suggested in your action plan, your symptoms don't get better.

- **Take your medication as prescribed:** Even if your asthma seems to be better, you should always get your doctor's consent before making any modifications to your treatment plan. Bringing your medications with you to every doctor's appointment is a smart idea. If you're taking your meds as prescribed and at the right dosage, your doctor can verify it.

- **Be mindful of use quick-relief inhalers more frequently:** Your asthma isn't under control if you find yourself depending on your albuterol or another type of quick-relief inhaler. Consult your physician to modify your treatment plan.

Prevention of COPD

In contrast to certain other illnesses, COPD usually has a known origin, a known course of therapy, and methods for delaying the disease's progression. Since cigarette smoking is directly linked to most cases of COPD, quitting smoking as soon as possible is the greatest approach to prevent the disease.

These straightforward suggestions could be challenging for long-term smokers to adhere to, particularly if they have made several unsuccessful attempts to stop smoking. But keep trying to stop nonetheless. Selecting a smoking cessation program that can assist you in quitting permanently is essential. This is your best opportunity to minimize lung damage.

Another risk factor for COPD is exposure to chemical fumes and dusts at work. Speak with your supervisor about the best ways to protect yourself, such as wearing respiratory protection equipment, if you work with these kinds of lung irritants.

The actions listed below can assist in preventing COPD-related issues:

- Give up smoking to lower your risk of lung cancer and heart disease.

- To lower your risk of contracting some infections, think about being vaccinated against pneumococcal pneumonia and the flu each year.

- If you feel depressed or hopeless, or if you suspect you may be depressed, consult a physician.

Prevention of Lung Cancer

Lung cancer cannot be completely prevented, but you can lower your risk by doing the following:

- **Avoid smoking:** Don't start smoking if you've never done it before. Have a conversation with your kids about quitting smoking so they may learn how to reduce their exposure to this significant risk factor for lung cancer.

- Talk to your kids about the risks of smoking from an early age so they can learn to say no to peer pressure.

- **Exercise Frequently:** If you don't currently work out often, begin cautiously. On most days of the week, try to work out.

- **Stop smoking:** Give up smoking right away. Even if you have smoked for a long time, quitting lowers your risk of developing lung cancer. Consult your physician about effective cessation products and techniques. Support groups, medicine, and nicotine replacement treatment are some of the options.

- **Steer clear of secondhand smoke:** Urge your smoking roommate or coworker to give up. Ask them to smoke outside, at the very least. Seek for smoke-free options and stay away from smoking venues, such as bars and restaurants.

- **Test your home for radon:** Check the radon levels in your house, especially if you reside in a region where the gas is known to be contaminated. Your home might be safer if the increased radon levels are corrected. Speak with the local section of the American Lung Association or the public health department for information on radon testing.

- **Eat lots of fruits and vegetables:** Pick a diet high in a variety of fruits and vegetables and well-balanced. Food is the best way to get vitamins and other minerals. Vitamin tablets in large dosages should be avoided as they may be harmful. For example, researchers supplemented heavy smokers with beta-carotene to lower the risk of lung cancer. The results indicated that smokers' risk of cancer was elevated by the supplements.

- **Steer clear of carcinogens at work:** Take safety measures to shield yourself from hazardous chemical exposure at work. Following your employer's instructions, take action. If you are provided a face mask for protection, for example, wear it at all times. What other precautions can you take to keep yourself safe at work? To learn more, speak with your doctor. Smoking raises the possibility that lung damage from occupational carcinogens will occur.

Prevention of Pneumonia

To lessen the risk of pneumonia:

- **Get vaccinated:** There are vaccinations available to protect against some strains of the flu and pneumonia. See your doctor if you intend to receive these injections. Even if you remember getting vaccinated against pneumonia in the past, the recommendations for vaccines have changed, so be sure to check with your doctor to find out your current immunization status.

- **Ensure that kids receive their vaccines**: For children under two years old and those between the ages of two and five who are more vulnerable to pneumococcal illness, doctors advise getting a separate pneumonia vaccination. Children enrolled in group daycare facilities must also receive the vaccination. Immunization against influenza is also advised by doctors for children older than six months.

- **Eat Healthy:** Alcohol-based hand sanitizers can aid in preventing respiratory infections, which can occasionally result in pneumonia. Hands-wash frequently.

- **Steer clear of smoking:** Smoking weakens the natural defenses your lungs have against respiratory illnesses.

- **Keep your immune system strong:** Eat a balanced diet, undertake regular exercise, and get enough rest.

Prevention of Pulmonary Embolism

One method to protect yourself from pulmonary embolisms is to avoid clots in the deep veins of your legs. In order to reduce blood clots, the majority of hospitals implement preventative measures such as the ones listed below:

- **Anticoagulants:** Patients who are at risk of clotting are frequently prescribed these medications, both before and after surgery. In addition, if a patient has a specific medical condition—like a heart attack, stroke, or cancer-related issues—they are frequently given them upon admission to the hospital.

- **Compression stockings:** By gradually compressing the legs, compression stockings improve blood flow via the veins and muscles of the legs. They provide an easy, affordable, and safe means of preventing blood clots in the legs prior to, during, and following surgery.

- **Elevate your legs:** It can be quite helpful to elevate your legs whenever you can, especially at night. Using blocks or books, raise the foot of your bed by 4 to 6 inches (10 to 15 cm).

- **Physical activity:** By reducing the danger of a pulmonary embolism, moving as soon as possible following surgery aids in the healing process. For this primary reason, even if you are in discomfort at the site of your surgical incision, your nurse may still recommend that you walk on the day after your procedure.

- **pneumatic compression:** Thigh-high or calf-high cuffs that automatically inflate and deflate every few minutes are used in pneumatic compression therapy. Your legs' veins are compressed and massaged as a result, increasing blood flow.

Prevention while traveling

Blood clots are more likely to occur during long-distance travel, but they are not common. Speak with your healthcare practitioner if blood clot risk factors make you anxious about traveling.

Your physician might advise you to take the following steps to lessen the risk of blood clots when traveling:

- **Drink plenty of fluids:** The best liquid to avoid dehydration, which can result in the formation of blood clots, Is water. Steer clear of alcohol as it can cause dehydration.

- **Take a break from sitting:** Walk across the cabin of the airplane about once every hour. While driving, occasionally pull over and do a few laps around the vehicle. Bend your knees deeply a few times.

- **Adjust your seat:** Every fifteen to thirty minutes, raise your toes and move your ankles in circles.

- **Wear support stockings:** They might be suggested by your doctor to help with circulation and fluid movement in your legs. Compression stockings come in a variety of fashionable hues and textures. Stocking butlers are devices that assist you in pulling on your stockings.

Prevention of Tuberculosis

You might need to take medication to treat the active TB disease if your test results indicate that you have a latent TB infection.

Preventing the spread of disease

If you have active tuberculosis, you will need to look after other people in order to avoid infection. For four, six, or nine months, you will take medication. Throughout the entire procedure, take all prescribed drugs as instructed.

The TB bacteria can spread to other people during the first two to three weeks. Use the following precautions to keep people safe:

- Stay inside.
- Spend as little time as possible with your family and isolate yourself at home. Take a nap in a different room.
- Open doors to let in some fresh air. The TB bacteria spreads more readily in small areas. Open the windows if the outside temperature is not too low. Use a fan to get the air out. Use one fan to pull air in and another to push it out of any windows that are open.
- If you must interact with people, put on a mask. Request that the other family members don masks for their own protection.
- Every time you sneeze or cough, cover your mouth with a tissue. Once the soiled tissue has been placed in a bag, close it and discard it.

Vaccinations

Babies who receive the bacilli Calmette-Guerin (BCG) vaccine are frequently given this injection in nations where tuberculosis is endemic. Little children who are more susceptible to acquiring active tuberculosis in the fluid surrounding their brains and spinal cords are shielded by this.

The vaccine might not offer protection against lung diseases, which are more common in the United States. Numerous novel tuberculosis vaccines are under development and testing at different phases.

Prevention of Influenza (FLU)

For everyone six months of age or older, the U.S. Centers for Disease Control and Prevention (CDC) advises being vaccinated against the flu each year. Having a flu shot may reduce your chance of becoming ill. Should the virus cause a serious illness, receiving the flu shot reduces your chances of needing hospitalization. The flu vaccination also reduces the chance of influenza-related death.

Given that coronavirus disease and the flu share similar symptoms, vaccination against the flu is necessary. It's likely that COVID-19 and the virus are spreading simultaneously. The most effective prevention against both is vaccination.

Additionally, you can frequently receive both the COVID-19 and flu vaccines in a one visit if you schedule both at the same time.

The four influenza viruses that are anticipated to be most prevalent during this flu season are all protected against by this year's seasonal flu vaccines. The vaccination will be offered as a nasal spray and an injection this year. Additionally, high-dose influenza vaccinations will be available to those 65 years of age and above.

The nasal spray is advised for use in the age range of 2 to 49. It is not advised for some groups, including:

- those who previously have a severe adverse reaction to a flu vaccine.
- expectant women.

- Children taking aspirin or a medication containing salicylate who are 17 years of age or younger.
- those with compromised immune systems, as well as those who support or are in close proximity to those who do.
- Children with a diagnosis of asthma or wheeze during the last 12 months, between the ages of 2 and 4.
- people who just had treatment for their sickness with antiviral medication.
- individuals who, as in the case of a cochlear implant, either currently have or may develop a CSF leak in the future.

It is still possible to receive the flu shot if you are allergic to eggs.

Controlling the spread of infection

Considering the shortcomings of the influenza vaccine, it's critical to take more precautions to stop the virus from spreading, such as:

- **Regular Handwashing:** Wash your hands with soap and water for at least 20 seconds, being sure to wash them again. Use an alcohol-based hand sanitizer that contains at least 60% alcohol if soap and water are not readily available. Ensure that your loved ones and regular company are aware of the need of hand washing. This is particularly relevant to the younger ones.

- **Avoid touching your face:** You can prevent germs from entering your mouth, nose, or eyes by keeping your hands out of those regions.
- **Cover your coughs and sneezes:** Sneeze or cough into your elbow or a tissue. Next, give yourself a hand wash.
- **Clean surfaces:** Keep frequently touched surfaces clean to avoid transferring the virus to your face when you touch one infected surface and then another.

Avoid crowds. Anywhere people congregate, including as child care facilities, schools, businesses, auditoriums, and public transit, is a prime location for the virus to spread swiftly. You can reduce your chance of infection by staying away from crowds during the busiest flu season.

Furthermore, avoid being around sick people. In order to reduce your risk of spreading the illness to others, if you are ill, stay at home for at least 24 hours after your fever has subsided.

Chapter Four

Keeping your healthy lungs

Although your lungs are the main component of your respiratory system and are always in motion, you may not give them much thought. We take more than 23,000 breaths a day, and during that time, the lungs remove waste from our blood and add oxygen—a vital component of all living things—to the blood. Our ability to breathe diminishes with age, making it more difficult to perform this vital gas exchange. Nonetheless, there are steps you may do to protect and even expand your lung capacity.

- **Stop Smoking and Avoid Second-hand Smoke:** The quickest way to strengthen your lungs if you use tobacco products is to stop smoking. Breathing gets harder because smoking cigarettes narrows airways. Long-term smokers are more likely to develop COPD, which includes emphysema and chronic bronchitis, as well as lung cancer. It might also cause chronic lung inflammation or edema. Breathing in secondhand smoke can lead to a variety of other issues, including chronic diseases and respiratory infections. But as soon as you stop smoking, your body starts to heal the damage, and the longer you don't smoke, the less likely you are to become ill.

- **Stay Hydrated and Maintain Good Hygiene:** Your lungs are the sole organ that can help with metabolism, which is the process of using oxygen to transform food into energy. Your body needs fuel from food. You cannot get all the nutrients you require from a single diet. Drinking water can help to thin the mucus that clogs your airways and lungs, which will facilitate breathing. Dehydration, however, causes thicken and stickier mucus, which can make breathing more difficult all around and increase the likelihood that you will get sick or that your allergies will get worse.

- **Engage in Regular Exercises:** Your heart and lungs have to work harder during exercise in order to get more oxygen into your muscles. In addition to strengthening your heart, regular exercise also benefits your lungs. With time, as your body grows more adept at transferring oxygen from the bloodstream to the working muscles, breathlessness during physical exertion reduces.

- **Schedule Regular Check-ups:** Even if you are feeling healthy, schedule regular visits with your healthcare practitioner since this can help avoid disease. This is particularly true for lung problems, which can occasionally go undetected for a very long time. If you're having trouble breathing, you should notify your healthcare professional right away.

- **Avoid exposure to Air Outdoor Pollution**: Even if the air outside might be healthier than the air inside, there are still a lot of pollutants in the outdoors that might be bad for your health. Over thirty percent of Americans reside in areas with toxic outdoor air. The two most common and harmful forms of pollution are ozone and particle pollution. Check out our State of the Air Report to find out more about how to keep your family safe and the outdoor air quality in your neighborhood.

- **Improve indoor air quality**: Mold, radon, household chemicals, and secondhand smoke are just a few of the things that can significantly affect the quality of indoor air and damage your lungs. If you have a long-term lung condition, indoor air pollution is particularly dangerous. There are several ways to enhance the quality of the air in your home, some of which include dusting frequently, replacing air filters, and quitting smoking.

- **Practice deep breathing:** Numerous deep breathing exercises can strengthen your lungs and help you cope with stressful circumstances. The capacity and endurance of the lungs are enhanced by these breathing exercises. The voluntary intake and exhalation of air as well as the contraction of the inspiratory muscles may therefore both increases.

- **Be updated in your vaccinations**: Vaccination is the best line of defense against the spread of infectious respiratory diseases like RSV, COVID-19, influenza, and pneumococcal pneumonia. People contract these ailments from one another. Since vaccinations can help avoid serious illness, they are especially crucial for those with lung disease.

- **Maintain good hygiene**: Frequently washing your hands for at least 20 seconds will help ward off illness. If flowing water is not easily accessible, hand sanitizer is a backup option. By wearing a mask or avoiding social situations, you can reduce your chance of becoming ill or spreading diseases in areas with high infection rates.

Get screened for Lung Cancer: Because low-dose CT scans detect lung cancer before symptoms appear, they can prevent lung cancer deaths in high-risk individuals. It is not recommended that everyone have the test, so find out if you are eligible by consulting your healthcare provider.

The End

www.ingramcontent.com/pod-product-compliance
Lightning Source LLC
Chambersburg PA
CBHW070821280726
48660CB00017B/2378